Dash Diet

Learn To Live Healthier With These Simple Meal Prep Recipes For Blood Pressure Control And Hypertension

(A Groundbreaking Method For Increasing Energy And Lowering Blood Pressure)

JACQUES BOURASSA

TABLE OF CONTENT

The Advantages Of The Dash Diet For Enhancing Health

While it is true that the primary objective of the DASH diet is to mitigate hypertension, it is important to note that the diet imparts a myriad of health benefits that extend well beyond the mere reduction of elevated blood pressure levels. Consequently, health organizations and physicians highly endorse the DASH diet for a variety of individuals and purposes. While the primary objective of the DASH diet is to reduce elevated blood pressure levels or prevent the onset of hypertension, these advantages merely scratch the surface of the multitude of benefits that the DASH diet can afford individuals.

The DASH Diet is effective in reducing blood pressure
As previously elucidated in the preceding chapter, the conclusive iteration of the DASH diet has

demonstrated notable efficacy in alleviating hypertension. The efficacy of the diet in reducing elevated blood pressure can be attributed to its low sodium content and enhanced dietary fiber, along with the consumption of certain essential nutrients such as potassium and magnesium. The DASH diet not only demonstrates efficacy in reducing blood pressure, but its impact is nearly instantaneous.

If the DASH diet is followed, it is possible to observe a reduction in blood pressure by a few units within a span of two weeks. A decrease in blood pressure ranging between eight to fourteen units can exert a substantial influence on your health vulnerabilities in the span of months or years.

Evidently, the DASH diet is highly suitable for individuals with pre-existing hypertension or those exposed to high risk factors such as overweight, lifestyle factors, family medical history, or racial backgrounds that predispose them to hypertension.

The DASH Diet has the potential to inhibit or reverse the development of Metabolic Syndrome or Pre-diabetes.

Metabolic syndrome is commonly referred to as pre-diabetes due to its classification as a preceding condition to the onset of type 2 diabetes. Nonetheless, it should be noted that this is not an autonomous condition, but rather a conglomerate of diagnostic markers encompassing obesity, excessive abdominal adiposity, insulin insensitivity, elevated triglyceride and HDL cholesterol levels, as well as heightened fasting blood sugar levels.

The DASH diet is regarded as a highly effective dietary approach for individuals with metabolic syndrome due to various compelling reasons. Due to the diet's significant reduction in sugar content, adhering to this regimen will enhance your insulin sensitivity and contribute to the rectification of both excessive storage of abdominal fat and elevated blood sugar levels. The reduced consumption of unhealthy fats, coupled with an elevated intake of beneficial fats, will aid in the reduction of HDL cholesterol and triglyceride levels. Additionally, the diet can effectively address the issue of excess weight and abdominal fat associated with metabolic syndrome by virtue of its weight-loss benefits, particularly if one opts for a lower-calorie plan.

The Relationship between the DASH Diet and Type 2 Diabetes
In the event that you are diagnosed with type 2 diabetes or are deemed to have a considerable susceptibility to its onset, it is the professional advice of U.S. News & World Report to consider adhering to the DASH diet. The foods and principles of the DASH diet offer significant advantages to individuals with type 2 diabetes, as they share the same reasons why it is widely esteemed for its effectiveness in reversing metabolic syndrome. Nuts exhibit potential in stabilizing blood sugar levels and promoting glucose regulation in individuals with diabetes. Additionally, the inherent high-fiber composition of

nuts has the added benefit of reducing the rate at which sugar is absorbed into the bloodstream.

Weight loss is considered a highly significant advantage for individuals affected by type 2 diabetes, or those with an elevated susceptibility to acquiring the condition. The presence of surplus adipose tissue, particularly in the abdominal region, significantly contributes to a decline in insulin sensitivity. Furthermore, it augments the likelihood of experiencing heart disease, a risk that individuals with diabetes are already predisposed to.

The Impact of the DASH Diet on Cardiovascular Health

Individuals diagnosed with type 2 diabetes, metabolic syndrome, and hypertension are significantly more prone to the onset of cardiovascular disease. Given that the DASH diet has the potential to enhance or mitigate such conditions, it serves as an exceptional dietary regimen for the prevention of heart disease. Cardiovascular disease is the primary factor contributing to mortality rates in the United States, and a significant proportion of cases can be attributed to an unhealthy dietary pattern. The conventional American dietary pattern is characterized by inadequate consumption of dietary fiber and beneficial fats, and an excess intake of calories, unhealthy fats, and processed food products. The reason why the DASH diet has garnered the endorsement of AHA is because it encompasses all the essential elements of a diet that promotes heart health.

The DASH Diet Enhances General Well-being

The DASH diet is aligned with the findings of esteemed research on promoting holistic well-being and mitigating disease risks via dietary practices. Shedding pounds while following the DASH diet is an excellent ancillary benefit, however, it is important not to overlook the profound influence this dietary regimen exerts on your longevity and overall well-being. The DASH diet has garnered the approval and endorsement of esteemed medical professionals in the nation due to its comprehensive approach in addressing various pivotal health issues. When undertaking the DASH diet with the aim of weight reduction, it is crucial to bear in mind that weight loss is merely a favorable ancillary outcome of the diet. Nevertheless, you ought to be further pleased by the astounding potential for significant enhancements to both the quality and duration of your life.

Weight Reduction with the DASH Diet
The dietary plan prescribed by the DASH diet incorporates numerous elements recognized for their efficacy in promoting secure and sustainable weight reduction, making it an optimal option for individuals seeking to shed excess pounds, irrespective of their blood pressure levels. Due to the highly beneficial nature of the DASH diet, it is strongly recommended to adopt and adhere to this dietary approach throughout one's lifetime. This dietary plan does not offer a superficial solution,

nor does it pose any risks or dangers to your body when adhered to for an extended duration. This implies that as you experience the benefits of shedding weight, you can derive satisfaction from the knowledge that your endeavors are positively impacting both your physique and overall well-being. Upon attaining your weight-loss objective, not only will you acquire a more slender physique, but your overall well-being will also be enhanced.

The DASH diet possesses three key elements that contribute to its effectiveness in facilitating weight loss, apart from calorie monitoring: prioritizing the consumption of nourishing fats while abstaining from unhealthy fats, elevating fiber consumption, and ensuring a substantial intake of vitamin C and other essential nutrients.

The Fat Composition of the DASH Diet" "The Lipid Profile of the DASH Diet" "The DASH Diet's Lipid Content

By following the DASH diet, you will consequently reduce consumption of the unhealthy fats that are commonly prevalent in the typical American dietary patterns. Trans fats and unhealthy saturated fats are subject to strict limitations or even exclusion, while the inclusion of beneficial fats, such as plant-derived saturated fats and omega-3 fats, is significantly increased compared to the conventional American diet. Not only is this beneficial for cardiovascular health, but it also contributes to waistline management.

Typically, food items that contain considerable amounts of unhealthy fats, such as fast food and heavily processed foods, generally possess a substantial caloric value while lacking in nutritional quality. The DASH diet places an emphasis on consuming whole foods, providing the necessary fulfillment and nourishment without the presence of excessive empty calories.

The Fiber Composition of the DASH Diet

A diet rich in dietary fiber is not only beneficial for your overall health but also contributes positively to weight management. The DASH diet features a wide array of delectable foods that are abundant in soluble and insoluble fiber. This aids in fostering a sense of contentment, enhancing digestive processes, and decelerating the assimilation of dietary lipids and carbohydrates. This indicates a reduction in the accumulation of new fat in the abdominal region and a decrease in instances of elevated blood sugar levels, thereby resulting in a diminished inclination towards consuming carbohydrates and unhealthy foods.

The Vitamin C Composition of the DASH Diet
Due to the inclusion of delectable and nutritionally dense fresh produce in the DASH diet, individuals can acquire an ample supply of imperative vitamins, minerals, and a diverse array of antioxidants. Vitamin C holds significant importance in facilitating your weight-loss endeavors. In recent years, research

has demonstrated that Vitamin C plays a crucial role in eradicating accumulated fat and inhibiting hormonal responses that contribute to the deposition of adipose tissue in the abdominal region.

Vitamin C is diminished by a multitude of factors, with chronic stress emerging as one of the primary influences. Insufficient levels of vitamin C can indicate to the brain a state of stress, triggering the subsequent secretion of cortisol, which is a stress hormone. The role of cortisol is to accumulate fat in the abdominal region as a form of precaution against potential periods of food scarcity. While stress may not exert the same effect as it did in earlier times, it is perceived by your body through a similar lens.

By decreasing the level of stress in your life, you simultaneously diminish the quantity of cortisol being released into your circulatory system. The complete eradication of stress may not be attainable for the ordinary individual, however, ensuring an adequate intake of vitamin C can effectively mitigate its impact and restore the optimal balance of released cortisol. A decrease in cortisol levels translates to a reduction in the accumulation of new fat deposits. Furthermore, it signals your body to recognize that the existing reserves of fat are no longer necessary. The role of vitamin C becomes significant at this stage as well.

Vitamin C is an essential constituent of an inherent compound known as L-carnitine. L-carnitine is occasionally referred to as the fat-transporting compound, as it plays a significant role in the transportation of stored fat to sites within the body where it can be metabolized into glucose and subsequently utilized as an energy source.

Our physical organisms naturally synthesize L-carnitine, yet they depend on an adequate intake of vitamin C to enable this process. Our anatomical systems allocate primary preference to the utilization of vitamin C at any given point. The foremost objective is to utilize it in combating infection and regenerating cells. Any remaining quantity may be utilized for the production of L-carnitine.

The issue lies in the fact that vitamin C is a water-soluble nutrient, leading to its predominant excretion through urine, while only a minute fraction is retained in our bodies. This is precisely why ensuring a sufficient daily intake of vitamin C is imperative for the purpose of reducing body fat. The DASH diet tackles this issue by incorporating a substantial amount of fresh produce, specifically those that are abundant in vitamin C. In addition to facilitating the burning of stored fat, you will also provide a much-needed enhancement to your immune system.

The DASH diet employs these factors to facilitate safe and comfortable weight loss while promoting your overall well-being. It further employs a rational yet manageable calorie intake with the aim of aiding you in achieving your objectives. This segment of the DASH diet can be fully tailored based on individual preferences, objectives, and specific caloric requirements.

Does The Dash Diet Live Up To Its Acclaimed Reputation?

Among various aspects, the DASH diet typically provides education and guidance to individuals with hypertension, with the intention of mitigating the detrimental consequences of elevated blood pressure. By adhering to the DASH diet, it is conceivable that the incidence of cardiovascular disorders, cerebrovascular accidents, and renal lithiasis is mitigated to a controllable extent.

Advantages Offered by the DASH Diet

Multiple studies conducted by health researchers have provided evidence suggesting that individuals with hypertension can effectively manage their blood pressure by adhering to the recommendations outlined in the Dietary Approaches to Stop Hypertension (DASH) diet. Elevated blood pressure is a predominant contributor to global mortality rates.

Additionally, elevated blood pressure is also a significant factor in the increased prevalence of diabetes, cardiovascular conditions, and osteoporosis

These illnesses present a significant challenge in terms of treatment due to their chronic nature. The DASH diet, in light of this rationale, promotes preventive measures as opposed to treatment, which may be unattainable for certain individuals due to the exorbitant price of medications.

Elevated levels of cholesterol in the bloodstream can be detrimental to one's overall well-being. This is due to its role in the promotion of vascular thickening, thereby posing a potential threat to human life.

The DASH diet incorporates low-cholesterol or cholesterol-free foods. The inclusion of fruits, low-fat dairy products, and vegetables in the DASH diet has been documented to effectively reduce the risk of developing hypertension over an extended period.

A number of foods included in the Dietary Approaches to Stop Hypertension (DASH) regimen possess the ability to effectively lower the sodium concentrations within the human body.

Numerous health professionals recommend that, in routine conditions, the optimal daily intake of sodium for a healthy human body is 2400 mg. In comparison to conventional dietary choices, the sodium content can potentially reach a level of 3500 mg in this particular context, which is regarded as potentially detrimental, particularly in relation to blood pressure regulation.

Elevated sodium levels are a significant factor in the increase of blood pressure, thereby leading to hypertension. Failure to address this condition may ultimately culminate in fatality.

In addition to addressing hypertension concerns, the DASH diet offers a significant amount of dietary fiber, which effectively supports gastrointestinal health and promotes smooth digestion within the gastric system. Efficient digestion entails the adequate absorption of essential nutrients into the body's system, resulting in heightened energy levels and consequent increased fat metabolism.

When the levels of accumulated fats are diminished, there is a significant likelihood that the individual will eventually decrease their excessive weight. Hence, the DASH diet proves to be superior in comparison to the conventional diet.

Ultimately, individuals who typically experience inflammation of bodily tissues, particularly the cardiovascular system, stand to benefit from adhering to the DASH diet. The DASH diet exhibits relatively reduced levels of cholesterol. Elevated cholesterol levels lead to the thickening of blood vessels, resulting in diminished efficacy, as oxygen-rich blood may not adequately circulate to various bodily regions. An individual afflicted with thickened blood vessels commonly exhibits signs of fatigue due to inadequate oxygen circulation throughout the body. Due to this rationale, the DASH diet is particularly recommended for hypertensive patients as a means to increase their longevity.

What options are available to me in terms of food?
The Dash Diet includes a significant amount of fruits, vegetables, and grains in its composition. With that being noted, it contains a significant quantity of fiber, which aids in maintaining regular bowel movements. In order to acclimate your body to this dietary plan, gradually elevate the portions.
* A recommended intake of 4 - 5 servings of fruits, which provide a good source of dietary fiber, potassium, magnesium, vitamins, and minerals. An assortment of fruits including apples, bananas, berries, grapes, citrus fruits such as lemon and lime, pears, and pineapple.

* 4 – 5 Portions of vegetables - Additionally abundant in dietary fiber and essential vitamins. Some alternative ways to express the same thing in a formal tone could be: 1. The list comprises of artichokes, bell peppers, broccoli, cabbage, carrots, cauliflower, corn, green beans, mushrooms, lettuce, onions, potatoes, sprouts, and squash. 2. Included in the inventory are artichokes, bell peppers, broccoli, cabbage, carrots, cauliflower, corn, green beans, mushrooms, lettuce, onions, potatoes, sprouts, and squash. 3. The assemblage consists of artichokes, bell peppers, broccoli, cabbage, carrots, cauliflower, corn, green beans, mushrooms, lettuce, onions, potatoes, sprouts, and squash. 4. Contained within the assortment are artichokes, bell peppers, broccoli, cabbage, carrots, cauliflower, corn, green beans, mushrooms, lettuce, onions, potatoes, sprouts, and squash. 5. Among the items listed are artichokes, bell peppers, broccoli, cabbage, carrots, cauliflower, corn, green beans, mushrooms, lettuce, onions, potatoes, sprouts, and squash.

Allocating a recommended daily intake of 2-3 portions of low-fat dairy will fulfill your body's calcium, protein, and vitamin D requirements. Low-fat cheeses, curds, skim milk, plant-based spreads, reduced-fat cream, and non-fat yogurt. Priority is given to low-fat or fat-free options.

* A maximum of 6 portions of lean meat, fish, or poultry can be consumed, as they are abundant in proteins, zinc, and B vitamins. Beef, poultry (including chicken and turkey), eggs, seafood (comprising fish, salmon, and shrimp).

**2 to 3 Portions of oils and fats - These fats are essential for the absorption of vitamins and nutrients. The recommended portion size may consist of one tablespoon. low-fat mayonnaise, a tsp. consisting of margarine and a quantity of two tablespoons. of lite salad dressings.

* Consume 4 - 5 portions of legumes, nuts, and seeds, as these foods supply ample amounts of protein, magnesium, potassium, fiber, and phytochemicals. Almonds, peanuts, pistachios, legumes, and pulses.

* A recommended daily intake of grains is 6-8 servings. Examples of suitable grains include barley, brown rice, oats, whole wheat bread, whole wheat tortillas, whole wheat pasta, whole grain cereal, and wild rice.

Guidelines for the Dash Diet

Do refrain from extending your hand towards the salt.
Please stow it if it is present on your dining table. I acknowledge that, for me, it constituted the initial and most challenging task. Although it may appear amusing to certain individuals, I had developed a customary practice of incorporating salt into nearly all of my culinary creations. Alternatively, opt for the utilization of herbs and spices devoid of sodium in order to add flavor to your culinary preparation.
Make sure to incorporate a generous amount of vegetables and whole grains into your diet.
Abundant in dietary fiber, protein, potassium, and calcium. Consuming an ample quantity of these items will

effectively reduce and maintain a healthy blood pressure level.

Refrain from indulging in confections.

While it is not necessary to completely forsake them, it is advisable to exercise restraint. Opt for fat-free or low-fat options. Fruit will effectively quell your cravings for sweetness.

Please restrict the quantity of meat consumed.

Reduce your daily consumption to a maximum of a few servings if you are currently exceeding that amount. Even lean cuts of meat may contain levels of fat and cholesterol, therefore it is advisable not to primarily base your dietary choices on such sources.

Please exercise caution and moderation when consuming alcoholic beverages.

Excessive consumption of alcohol can elevate blood pressure levels. Please restrict your consumption to a maximum of one or two per day, if any at all.

Please ensure that you transition to a new dietary regimen in a gradual manner.

Gradually include portions of fruits, vegetables, and whole grains into your diet to mitigate the risk of experiencing gastrointestinal discomfort such as diarrhea or bloating, particularly if you are unaccustomed to consuming a fiber-rich regimen.

Don't give up.

If you require assistance, avail yourself of it. Adhering to a dietary regimen may prove challenging for certain individuals. It is advisable to consult with your physician or a registered dietitian, as they can offer valuable recommendations to facilitate compliance with the prescribed diet.

Do add physical activity.

Please take into account your level of physical activity in conjunction with the Dash Diet. When both are combined, there is a higher probability of reducing blood pressure and achieving weight loss.

Tips for Dining Out

Avoid binge eating.

Do not consider dining out as a form of respite from maintaining a nutritious diet. Instead, dedicate yourself to selecting more nutritious options when ordering meals. Should you have the inclination to partake in excess, kindly endeavor to either distribute it amongst those present at the dining table or make arrangements to carry a portion of it back to your place of residence.

Don't go starving.

Abstaining from eating in order to make space can result in excessive consumption. Kindly ensure to partake in a small sustenance prior to venturing outdoors.

Research.

Many restaurants have embraced the digital sphere in recent times. Conduct a search to locate and review their menu in advance.

Portion Control.

Indulging in food until you have satisfied your hunger and possibly more, such is the mindset for those who are averse to food wastage. Alternatively, opt for a reduced portion such as an appetizer, engage in food-sharing with your dining companion, or consider the option of taking any leftovers with you.

Take your time.

Engaging in excessive consumption without restraint will result in your brain being unable to promptly signal satiety. Consume your food leisurely, savor the flavors, and you will be less prone to indulging excessively.

Do not hesitate to seek clarification.

Kindly request them to ensure that your meal is prepared without the addition of salt.

Please request that sauces and dressings be served separately.

Kindly opt for replacing the fried side dishes with the choice of either steamed vegetables or a salad.

Limit or avoid.

Smoked, or pickled foods.

Ketchup, barbeque sauce, pickles, as well as soy and teriyaki sauces, along with salad dressings, should be avoided due to their elevated sodium content.

Added sugar.

Watch what you drink.

Alcohol possesses negligible nutritional value but is abundant in caloric content. Limit your consumption. Men are advised to consume two capsules per day, while women are recommended to consume one capsule per day.

Select from the options of water, club soda, tea, or fruit juice. Coffee is acceptable, but it is advisable to opt for decaffeinated alternatives, as the caffeine content has the potential to temporarily elevate blood pressure.

Oats With A Tasty Combination Of Banana And Nuts

- 2 bananas, peeled and mashed
- 1 tsp. vanilla extract
- 2 tbsp. chia seeds
- 1 cup almond milk
- ¼ cup walnuts, chopped
- 2 cups water
- 1 cup oats, steel-cut

Combine the water, oats, milk, walnuts, chia seeds, bananas, and vanilla in a cooking pot.

Thoroughly blend and simmer the mixture over a moderate heat.

Allow the mixture to simmer, while stirring at regular intervals, for a duration of 15 minutes.

Proceed to transfer the contents into your designated serving bowls and present them while still warm.

What Does The Term 'Dash Diet' Signify?

When it pertains to obtaining a comprehensive understanding of the DASH Diet, there are several key factors that necessitate careful examination. As you are likely aware, the dietary choices we make have a significant impact on our overall state of health. Hence, a dietary regimen containing harmful components such as cholesterol and saturated fats is indisputably linked to the development of hypertension and a myriad of other life-threatening ailments. Nevertheless, the ingestion of appropriate dietary choices can reduce the likelihood of developing these grave health conditions. There exists a specialized dietary regimen specifically devised to mitigate elevated blood pressure levels, commonly referred to as hypertension. This specific dietary regimen is commonly known as the DASH Diet.

What is the gist of the matter?

The clinical studies conducted by researchers from the NHBL institute have led to the recommendation of the DASH Diet. Upon meticulous analysis and rigorous experimental evaluation, the researchers arrived at the finding that an alimentary regimen containing ample amounts of magnesium, potassium, calcium, dietary fiber, and protein yields remarkable reductions in elevated blood pressure levels. Moreover, the research substantiated the notion that adhering to a diet rich in fruits and vegetables, while minimizing fat consumption, can significantly diminish the likelihood of developing hypertension. Additionally, the diet provides expedient outcomes with minimal time investment.

The DASH diet emphasizes three primary components, namely magnesium, potassium, and calcium.

These nutrients have been acknowledged for their ability to decrease elevated blood pressure levels. According to a research report, a typical 2000 calorie diet contains approximately 500 milligrams of magnesium, 1.2 grams of calcium, and 4.7 grams of potassium.

Using the DASH Diet

Utilizing and adhering to a DASH diet is quite uncomplicated and direct, as it requires minimal time for meal preparation. In addition to abstaining from foods that are rich in cholesterol, the dieter is urged to enhance their consumption of vegetables, grains, and fruits to the greatest extent feasible. Taking into account that the foods comprising the DASH diet contain a significant amount of dietary fiber, it is highly recommended that you progressively increase the incorporation of fiber-rich foods into your diet as a preventive measure against digestive complications and diarrhea. In addition, you may enhance your fiber intake by incorporating an additional portion of fruits and vegetables into your dietary regimen.

Grains, B vitamins, and minerals are all excellent sources of dietary fiber. For example, alternative grain products such as whole grains, bran, wheat breads, wheat germ, and low-fat cereals can be incorporated into your diet to increase your fiber intake.

It is essential to examine the labels of packaged and processed foods to ascertain their constituent elements. Select food items that are characterized by their low levels of cholesterol, saturated fats, sodium, chocolates, and similar substances. For those seeking to consume meat, it is advisable to restrict their daily consumption to no more than six ounces. Additionally, skim milk or low-fat milk can serve as an alternative protein source.

The DASH diet has gained significant traction among individuals mindful of their health, primarily due to its lack of reliance on specialized recipes and meals. There are no specific limitations with regards to calorie monitoring and meal preparations, provided that one abstains from consuming foods that are rich in cholesterol and saturated fats. The DASH diet regimen is a nutritious eating plan that focuses on the three crucial minerals known to have a positive impact on elevated blood pressure.

Almond Muffins

Ingredients

- 2 tsp grated lemon zest
- 2 Tbsp balsamic vinegar
- 2 Tbsp whole milk
- 3/4 cup extra-virgin olive oil
- 2/3 cup sliced almonds, toasted and crushed
- 1 3/4 cups all-purpose flour
- 2 tsp baking powder
- ½ tsp salt
- 1 cup sugar
- 4 large eggs
- 2 tsp grated orange zest

Directions

Preheat oven to 350°F. Insert paper liners into a muffin pan with a capacity of 12 cups.

Combine the flour, baking powder, and salt in a bowl, stirring to mix. In a bigger container, vigorously whisk the sugar,

Whisk the eggs and zest until they achieve a pale and fluffy consistency. Incorporate vinegar and milk into the mixture, and gradually blend in the oil using a beating motion. Combine

Combine the flour mixture and mix gently by hand until fully incorporated. Add almonds. Fill the liners nearly up to the brim.

Bake until a golden hue is achieved, for a duration of 20 to 25 minutes. Allow the dish to cool in the pan for a duration of 10 minutes. Put muffins on wire

Allow the dish to rest for an additional 5 minutes on a cooling rack.

The Dash Diet's Benefits

The benefits of the DASH diet surpass the reduction of blood pressure and prevention of heart-related illnesses.

Regulating blood pressure: The measurement of blood pressure within the human body encompasses the exertion of force on our blood vessels and organs during the circulation of blood. When the blood pressure surpasses a designated threshold, it can lead to a range of organ abnormalities, such as the occurrence of heart failure.

Blood pressure is assessed through two components: systolic pressure, which corresponds to the pressure exerted in the blood vessels during heart contractions, and diastolic pressure, which represents the pressure exerted in the blood vessels during the heart's resting phase. Generally, individuals in the adult population typically possess a systolic blood pressure below 120 mmHg and a diastolic pressure below 80 mmHg. Those surpassing these thresholds are categorized as having elevated blood pressure.

The DASH diet effectively reduces blood pressure levels by restricting salt intake and prioritizing the consumption of vegetables, healthy fats, lean proteins, and fruits. Indeed, a reduction in salt intake directly correlates with a decrease in blood pressure. The proficient implementation of the DASH diet has the potential to decrease systolic blood pressure by an average of 12 mm Hg and diastolic blood pressure by 5 mm Hg.

The DASH diet not only caters to individuals with hypertension, but it may also yield advantageous outcomes for individuals with regular blood pressure levels. The task at hand is to consume satisfactory amounts of sodium while abiding by the nutritional guidelines of the DASH diet.

lose weight:
Individuals who exhibit hypertension are recommended to actively control their body weight, as an excessive amount of weight can potentially give

rise to various health complications. The coexistence of obesity and elevated blood pressure can potentially lead to cardiac and organ dysfunction. The DASH diet has the potential to assist individuals in decreasing their blood pressure while concurrently achieving weight loss. This can be attributed to the nourishing meals recommended in the DASH diet. To promote weight loss, it is advised for individuals to decrease their daily consumption of calories.

Moreover, the DASH diet has exhibited evidence of additional health advantages:

Mitigates the possibility of cancer: individuals adhering to the DASH dietary regimen experience a diminished likelihood of developing colorectal and breast cancer.

It assesses metabolic syndrome: The dietary regimen reduces the likelihood of acquiring metabolic syndrome.

The management of diabetes involves the implementation of highly advantageous dietary plans, particularly for individuals diagnosed with type 2 diabetes.

Cardiovascular Disease: The diet mitigates the likelihood of developing cardiovascular disease and experiencing a stroke.

Classification Of Nutritional Categories Within The Dash Dietary Approach

The Dash diet will prove to be convenient to adhere to, as it incorporates readily available food items that can be easily procured at your nearby grocery store. The Dash diet proposes recommended daily servings for each of the food groups. The quantity of portions you can consume is contingent upon your daily caloric requirements.

1. Water. In order to ensure optimal nutrient intake, it is imperative to maintain adequate hydration on a daily basis, as this plays a significant role in promoting optimal bodily functions. It is imperative to prevent dehydration by ensuring adequate consumption of

water to maintain optimal hydration levels of your vital organs.

Dangers of Dehydration. The human adult physique comprises approximately 60 to 70 percent water. The lean tissue possesses a greater capacity for water retention in comparison to adipose tissue. In the event of being overweight, your body faces increased difficulty in retaining the necessary amount of water vital for facilitating the proper functioning of your essential organs.

If one becomes dehydrated, it can disrupt the overall circulation of fluids throughout the entire body. This particular action results in the reduction of blood pressure as it diminishes the blood flow, leading to a decrease in the pressure exerted by the blood against the walls of the arteries. This diminishes the oxygen content in the bloodstream, leading to a decrease in the oxygen supply to crucial organs and bodily tissues. Insufficient hydration will result in an overall imbalance within your body.

The volume of water present in your body is reduced as a result of processes such as urine production, bowel movements, sweat evaporation, and respiration. This is the reason why it is crucial to restore your water reservoir through the consumption of food and beverages that are rich in water content.

2. Enriched breakfast cereal, pasta, rice, and baked goods. Opting for whole grain options within this food category is highly recommended. They shall furnish you with the utmost nutrients, along with elevated levels of vitamins and minerals. Furthermore, they possess minimal quantities of processed substances such as dyes and added sugars.

3. Vegetables & Fruits. When making selections of fruits and vegetables, it is advisable to opt for a diverse range of hues. The greater the vibrancy of the colors, the higher the nutritional content they possess.

4. Milk, Yogurt, and Cheese. Dairy plays a crucial role in numerous physiological processes within the human body. It serves as an excellent calcium source, a mineral essential for the proper functioning of all bodily processes.

Calcium derived from dairy consumption facilitates the development of robust dental and skeletal structures, aids in the effective transmission of neural signals, contributes to muscular relaxation and contraction, plays a role in the synthesis and release of pivotal hormones and biochemicals within the body, and ensures the sustenance of a regular cardiac rhythm.

5. Seafood, Poultry, Legumes, and Tree Nuts. This particular food category provides the body with essential nutrients such as iron, zinc, protein, vitamin B, enhancing overall health and strength. Ensure that you select lean portions of meat and eliminate the skin from poultry such as turkey, chicken, and other poultry varieties.

6. Fats, Oils, Sweets, Supplements. It is recommended that you incorporate calcium, vitamin D, and vitamin B12 into your daily routine by means of additional supplements in order to meet the specific nutritional requirements. Exercise careful discretion when selecting your oils. Prominent sources of oil include coconut oil and extra-virgin olive oil.

Ways To Adhere To The Dietary Approaches To Stop Hypertension (Dash) Protocol Useful Tips

Adjusting to the DASH diet does not present a formidable challenge. To initiate the process, employ the subsequent approaches. Gradually initiate the process, refraining from attempting an immediate overhaul of your lifestyle.

Consume a greater variety of fruits and vegetables
If you incorporate one or two servings of vegetables into your daily meals, consider augmenting your intake by adding an additional serving during both lunch and dinner.
If one refrains from consuming fruit or juice during breakfast, it is advisable to incorporate a fruit into subsequent meals or consume it as a mid-meal snack.

Frequently opt for dairy products that are either fat-free or low in fat.

Systematically augment the daily intake of dairy products. To provide an illustration, it is advisable to incorporate milk into your mid-morning or midday meal as an alternative to consuming carbonated beverages, alcoholic beverages, or sugary teas.

Decrease red meat intake.
Buy less meat.
Constrain the intake of meat to a maximum of 200 grams per day.
If one consumes substantial quantities of meat, it is advisable to gradually decrease the portion sizes, ideally by two or three increments.
Please incorporate at least two vegetarian meal options into the menu on a weekly basis.
To prepare casseroles and pies, try to use less meat and more vegetables, cereals and legumes

Refrain from consuming sodium, sugar (including beverages with high sugar content), and confectionaries, and make a conscious effort to minimize the use of salt in culinary preparations.

Incorporating herbs and spices into your culinary preparations can effectively reduce the sodium content of a dish, potentially resulting in its complete elimination.

Refrain from consuming foods that consist of saturated fat, cholesterol, or Trans fats.
Utilize a reduced quantity, equivalent to half of the standard measure, of butter, margarine, and salad flavoring. Butter and margarine can be effectively substituted with liquid oils.
Elevate the proportion of cereals, poultry, seafood, and nuts within your dietary intake.
Opt for whole grain products as they possess an abundance of nutrients, specifically B vitamins. Examples of such products include whole grain breads, cereals, and corn flakes.

You should restrict your alcohol consumption to a maximum of 2 drinks per day, and no more than 10 drinks per week.

Satisfy your craving for sweets with an assortment of fresh, dried fruits, or fruit preserves.

Cease the act of smoking, if you have not already done so. Smoking adversely affects the vascular system, leading to elevated blood pressure.

Always follow your weight. Achieving a weight that falls within the healthy range recommended for individuals of your age and gender will further decrease your blood pressure levels.

Check your blood pressure regularly.

If allocated, please ensure timely administration of your prescribed medications.

Please refer to the following recommended serving sizes for food groups in accordance with the DASH diet:

Recommended grain intake: 6-8 servings per day
This encompasses an assortment of food items such as bread, porridge, cereals, rice, and pasta. It serves as a highly

valuable source of both energy and dietary fiber.

In order to enhance the nutritional content of your diet, it is advisable to opt for whole grain products instead of refined flour. This is because whole grain products are rich sources of fiber and essential trace elements, such as magnesium. Specifically, opt for brown rice as opposed to white pasta, whole meal alternatives instead of refined options, and whole grain bread rather than white bread. Select items that originate from cereals or those that are solely made from 100% wheat.

Cereals possess minimal fat content, therefore refrain from adulterating their nutritional value by excessively incorporating butter, cream, or cheese sauces.

Recommended daily consumption of vegetables: 4-5 servings

Vegetables, including tomatoes, carrots, and broccoli, are replete with plentiful dietary fiber, vitamins, and essential minerals like potassium and magnesium. And please bear in mind, refrain from considering them merely as supplementary elements to main courses - the combination of assorted vegetables holds the potential to constitute a delightful standalone dish.

Both fresh and frozen vegetables are equally beneficial for one's well-being. To optimize the advantages derived from canned vegetables, it is imperative to ensure the absence of any additional sodium.

To augment the proportion of vegetables incorporated into your daily dietary intake, employ imaginative strategies. For instance, during the preparation of beef stew, incorporate a reduced quantity of diced vegetables.

Consumption of fruits should consist of 4-5 servings per day.

Similar to vegetables, fruits are abundant in fiber, potassium, and magnesium, and are generally low in fat, with the exception of coconut and avocado.

To initiate your day with fruits, incorporate a serving of orange juice in your breakfast routine, include a wholesome snack comprising a segment of apple or orange during the course of the day, and ensure not to overlook the gratification of a fruit salad complemented by low-fat yogurt as an indulgent topping for dessert.

Whenever feasible, employ the utilization of peeled fruits that are suitable for consumption. Pare back the skin of apples, peaches, and various pit-containing fruits to infuse a distinct flavor into culinary preparations, while simultaneously enhancing their nutritional value with enriched fiber content and an array of essential micronutrients.

Consume 2-3 servings of dairy products that are low in fat or completely fat-free on a daily basis.

Milk, yogurt, cheese, along with other dairy products, represent the primary source of calcium, vitamin D, and protein. Nevertheless, it is advisable to opt for low-fat or completely fat-free alternatives when it comes to dairy products, given that such products tend to be high in fat content, which can potentially contribute to the progression of atherosclerosis.

If you encounter difficulty in digesting dairy products, it is not necessary to entirely eliminate them from your dietary intake. One is able to select dairy products that are free from lactose.

Low-fat frozen yogurt can act as a viable alternative to sugary treats; one can enhance its nutritional and sensory appeal by incorporating fresh fruits.

Consume a maximum of two servings per day of meat, poultry, and fish.

This food provides a commendable amount of protein, vitamin B, iron, and zinc. Nevertheless, it is important to note that even lean meat harbors a substantial quantity of fat and cholesterol. Therefore, it is advisable to exercise restraint when consuming meat from animals.

The DASH diet does not incorporate meat as a significant constituent of the dietary regimen. Please consider allocating your typical serving of meat into either three or two portions, and complement it with a side of vegetables.

Prior to preparing meat-based dishes, it is advisable to meticulously eliminate any skin or fat present. Subsequently, the meat should be subjected to the cooking methods of boiling, simmering, or grilling, preferably abstaining from frying it in a pan with the inclusion of butter.

Nuts, seeds, and legumes: Consume 4-5 servings per week.
Almonds, sunflower seeds, lentils, peas, beans, and various other foods falling under this category serve as excellent sources of essential nutrients such as magnesium, potassium, and protein. They additionally include a substantial amount of dietary fiber and phytochemicals which have the potential to mitigate the risk of certain tumors and cardiovascular ailments.
Nuts possess a considerable quantity of fat, albeit consisting of beneficial monounsaturated fatty acids. Nuts possess a high caloric content and thus consumption ought to be exercised with moderation. A suitable approach would

be to incorporate them into salads or sauces.

Food items derived from soy protein, such as tofu or soy meat, present a viable substitute to animal-based meats due to their comprehensive inclusion of essential amino acids.

Fats and oils: Recommended consumption of 2-3 servings per day.

Dietary fats serve as a crucial component necessary for the assimilation of vital vitamins, as they play a pivotal role in fostering the development of the immune system. Nevertheless, an excessive quantity of adipose tissue amplifies the susceptibility to cardiovascular ailments, diabetes, and obesity. The DASH diet enables the maintenance of a wholesome equilibrium by allocating approximately 27% of daily caloric consumption towards beneficial unsaturated fats.

Commence adopting wise consumer habits by cultivating the practice of perusing the details on product labels, opting for sauces, mayonnaise, and margarines that possess either negligible or nonexistent amounts of saturated fats and trans-fatty acids.

Sweets: it is advisable to restrict consumption to fewer than 5 servings per week.
Even when adhering to the DASH diet, it is permissible to consume minimal quantities of sweetened food.
Sweets that adhere to the dietary guidelines of the DASH diet ought to be devoid of fat, examples being sherbet or sorbet, fruit-based ice cream, jelly, or marmalade.
Artificial sweeteners, such as aspartame or sucralose, can satiate your craving for sugary tastes, yet one must bear in mind that their consumption should be moderated to sensible levels.

At first glance, it may appear simpler; however, it is advisable not to hastily draw hasty inferences. Merely adhering to dietary regulations and instructions does not provide adequate evidence of successfully implementing the DASH diet. In other terms, this pertains not solely to your dietary choices, but rather, primarily focuses on cultivating a healthier lifestyle. Engaging in regular physical activity and performing exercises is vital in safeguarding the well-being of your cardiovascular system and promoting heart health.

Grape Leaf Cigar

Ingredients:

1 cup of chosen, washed and drained rice tea

300 gr of duckling ground

40 new and tender grape leaves

2 sliced tomatoes

1 lemon

1/2 kg of lean muscle

1 medium onion sliced

1 clove of garlic

2 tbsp butter

Syrian salt and pepper (see below) to taste

Preparation:

20 g freshly ground black pepper

20 grams of ground cinnamon

50 gr freshly ground black pepper

Mix it up and save it to use as needed. Method of preparation:

Prepare the filling. First, make the broth. Incorporate the muscle, onion, garlic, one of the tablespoons of butter, salt, and pepper into a pan. Add 2 liters of water and allow to simmer for a duration of 2 hours. The broth should be strained, and the muscle should be shredded. Reserve the meat and stock.

Immerse the rice in water that has reached its boiling point, allowing it to rest for a duration of 30 minutes. Thoroughly drain, gently exerting pressure using your hands. Transfer the contents into a bowl and incorporate the duckling, along with 2 tablespoons of shredded muscle, 2 tablespoons of broth, and the remaining quantity of butter. Salt and pepper. Thoroughly combine all ingredients, ensuring they are well-incorporated, while refraining from engaging in any kneading.

Ride the cigarettes. Protract every grape leaf ensuring that the portion exhibiting the most verdant hue is oriented in a downward direction. Evenly distribute the filling along the central vein of the leaf, aiming for approximately one tablespoon per leaf. Securely enclose and flex the extremities.

Arrange grape leaves in a pan. Upon the foliage, resides the segmented tomatoes and the pulverized sinew. Place the cigarettes onto this stratum. Gently warm the stock that has been set aside and pour it into the pan while still hot. Place a plate on top of the pan to stabilize it. Place a lid on the container and reduce the heat to a low setting. Cook for a duration of one hour and thirty minutes at a low temperature, ensuring that the pan remains consistently on the heat source.

Subsequently, remove the cover and proceed to apply pressure to the lemon, allowing its juice to be dispensed evenly on the cigarettes. Once more, please cover the dish and allow it to cook for an additional hour. In the event that the water becomes excessively evaporated, supplement it with additional broth. Exercise caution when extracting the cigarettes and proceed to serve.

Easy Buckwheat Pancakes

Ingredients

1 tablespoon vegetable oil

½ cup milk

½ cup water

2 bananas

½ cup buckwheat flour

2 egg whites

1 tablespoon baking powder

½ cup all-purpose flour

1 tablespoon sugar

METHOD

Combine the milk and egg whites in a mixing bowl. Carefully incorporate the vegetable oil into the mixture in a gradual manner.

In a distinct bowl, amalgamate all the dehydrated constituents, excluding the bananas.

Incorporate the egg white mixture into the dry ingredients and whisk until thoroughly blended. Gradually incorporate water into the mixture while whisking until a uniform consistency is achieved.

Preheat a griddle pan on a medium heat setting. In order to ascertain whether the pan has reached the desired temperature, you may place a droplet of water onto its surface and observe for any audible sizzling. Should the water emit such a sound, it indicates that the pan is adequately heated and suitable for culinary preparations.

Take a measuring cup and pour an amount equivalent to ½ cup of pancake batter onto the pan. Please grill the pancake on each side for approximately 2 minutes, or until the edges acquire a slight browning and are cooked thoroughly. Proceed with cooking the remaining batter.

Partition the pancakes evenly into four portions; garnish with thinly sliced bananas prior to serving.

Frittata With Asparagus And Onions That Have Been Caramelized

Ingredients:

¼ c. of finely sliced fresh basil
6 big eggs
½ teaspoon salt, kosher
¼ c. and one tablespoon of grated parmesan cheese
For taste: Ground pepper, fresh

1 teaspoon of olive oil
1 medium thinly sliced onion
2 teaspoon of balsamic vinegar
2 c. (about 1 bunch) asparagus, cut it into 1" segments
3 green sliced onions

Preparation:

Preheat the broiler to a high temperature beforehand.

Warm the 10-12" pan to a moderate temperature. Add olive oil and onions to the pan, then sauté for approximately 5 minutes or until they become tender and acquire a light golden-brown color. Incorporate balsamic vinegar into the mixture, ensuring thorough blending with the onions. Subsequently, incorporate the asparagus along with two tablespoons. By submerging the asparagus in water and covering it, steam can be generated to cook the asparagus for a duration of 4 minutes.

Meanwhile, beat the eggs in a standard (medium-sized) bowl and incorporate ¼ cup. of the parmesan

(grated), ¼ tsp. Add the required quantity of kosher salt and a small amount of freshly ground pepper.

Add basil, green onion, and the remaining ¼ teaspoon. Add an appropriate amount of Kosher salt to the cooked asparagus and onions. Mix them well.

Incorporate the combination of beaten eggs with the sautéed onions and asparagus, briefly blend using a spatula, gently folding the cooked egg from the base to the surface. Please ensure to cook for a minimum of two minutes on medium heat.

Carefully place the pan beneath the broiler for an estimated duration of 3 minutes, or until a desirable level of browning is achieved.

Remove from the broiler and evenly distribute the remaining 1 tablespoon. Sprinkle a generous amount of parmesan cheese and allow it to rest for about 5 minutes. Transfer the frittata from the skillet onto a wooden cutting board, proceed to slice it into four equal portions, and then elegantly serve.

The Essentials Of The Dash Diet: Key Information You Should Be Aware Of

The consumption of food items can have a profound impact on our overall well-being. Consuming a diet rich in high cholesterol and saturated fats can lead to the development of elevated blood pressure and various other health complications. One can potentially reduce the risk of developing these diseases by adopting the appropriate dietary selections.

Hypertension or elevated blood pressure can be mitigated by adhering to a specific dietary regimen. The diet that goes by the name of Dietary Approaches to Stop Hypertension, also known as DASH, is being referred to here.

There is a growing demand among individuals for the acquisition of the DASH diet, in an effort to effectively reduce their blood pressure levels. Individuals who are in the initial stages of developing hypertension will be prescribed this dietary regimen. My apologies for any misunderstanding, but it seems like you're requesting an alternative way to express the same idea in a formal tone. Please find the revised statement below: "Cardiovascular events such as myocardial infarctions, cerebrovascular accidents, and ruptured aneurysms manifest as adverse outcomes ensuing from elevated blood pressure."

The dietary regimen places emphasis on grains such as oatmeal due to their capacity to reduce blood pressure levels. Due to the substantial amount of dietary fiber they contain, whole wheat products tend to have a positive impact on one's overall health. They are replete with essential nutrients that are pivotal for your overall state of wellness. It is also advisable to consume a dietary intake consisting of 4 or 5 portions of fruits and vegetables per day. It is advisable to limit your consumption exclusively to dairy products that are labeled as nonfat, such as nonfat milk, nonfat cheeses, and nonfat yogurts. It is feasible to achieve a 1% outcome, although the prevailing consensus among experts is to discourage such an approach. Poultry such as chicken, turkey, and similar lean meats are also authorized. By adhering to this proposed course of action, you will have the ability to manage your elevated blood pressure. Presented herewith is a faithful replication of the Dash diet.

The DASH diet regimen has proven to be highly effective in maintaining optimal blood pressure levels for a significant number of individuals. Individuals who necessitate this dietary regimen in order to mitigate severe consequences must rigorously comply with its guidelines. Exercise caution as the ramifications can result in fatality. Implementing a balanced diet and engaging in regular physical activity can contribute to the effective management of your hypertension. I genuinely trust that you have found the dash diet plan to be of great utility.

What is the definition or description of the DASH diet?

Clinical trials conducted by the National Heart, Lung, and Blood Institute paved the way for the inception of the DASH diet (NHLBI). The study indicates that adhering to diets rich in potassium, magnesium, calcium, protein, and fiber, while keeping fat and cholesterol intake at a minimum, can noticeably reduce elevated blood pressure levels.

The DASH diet is renowned for its effectiveness in lowering blood pressure and contributing to the prevention of heart disease, stroke, diabetes, and several types of cancers. Based on the study, it has been observed that the impacts of the DASH diet become evident within a fortnight of initiating the dietary regimen. Consuming a diet that is rich in vegetables, fruits, and low-fat dairy products has been proven to significantly reduce blood pressure levels.

TO WHOM DOES THE DASH DIET APPLY?

Incorporating a DASH (Dietary Approaches to Stop Hypertension) diet can be an essential element of any well-balanced dietary plan. It will facilitate the reduction of blood pressure and enhance cardiac well-being through the reduction of LDL cholesterol and inflammatory markers.

Magnesium, calcium, and potassium constitute pivotal constituents of the DASH diet. Such minerals might have potential benefits in managing hypertension. A standard 2,000-calorie diet would typically comprise of 500 milligrams of magnesium, 4.7 grams of potassium, and 1.2 grams of calcium.

How can the DASH diet be effectively implemented?

Consuming a diet low in sodium and rich in potassium, calcium, and magnesium, as part of a low-sodium dietary regimen, can effectively reduce blood pressure levels. The dietary regimen is rich in fiber, which contributes to the reduction of blood pressure and facilitates weight loss, thereby assisting in the decrease of blood pressure.

What types of foods are recommended on the DASH diet?

Whole grains such as whole wheat, brown rice, barley, oats, and quinoa have been found to reduce the risk of various ailments due to their high nutrient content. Nonetheless, processed grains are deficient in essential nutrients and should be abstained from.

Substitute full-fat dairy products with fat-free or low-fat options such as skim milk, low-fat yogurt, Greek yogurt, and low-fat paneer. Lactose-intolerant individuals have the alternative of consuming lactose-free milk and dairy products.

A significant component of a DASH-style diet entails the inclusion of various types of nuts, legumes, such as beans and lentils, as well as seeds like sunflower and melon seeds, among others. They possess substantial quantities of dietary fiber, protein, omega three fatty acids, vitamins, as well as essential minerals such as zinc and magnesium, among other nutrients. Nuts contain a significant amount of healthy fats, however, it is advisable to restrict consumption due to their elevated caloric density. Decrease your consumption of salt and sugar by abstaining from salt and honey roasted nuts.

It is advised to refrain from consuming foods that are high in saturated fat and instead opt for lean meats, eggs, poultry, and fish. It is imperative to maintain proper regulation of sodium levels in processed meats such as bacon, ham, sausages, and salami. Consumption of red meat should be limited to infrequent instances.

Incorporating vegetables into every meal is highly advisable. Potassium, a mineral found in fruits and vegetables, plays a crucial role in the reduction of blood pressure. Commence by establishing a basic objective and progressively advance if you do not possess an inclination towards consuming fruits and vegetables. Incorporate an additional fruit or vegetable into your daily dietary intake, in addition to those that you already consume. I find whole fruits to be more appealing than juices. Dried fruits, such as raisins, cranberries, figs, and various other varieties, could serve as a delightful choice for a journey on the road.

In order to ensure optimal health, it is advisable to limit the intake of saturated fats and total fats in one's diet. The presence of fats is beneficial for facilitating the absorption of fat-soluble vitamins and enhancing the body's ability to combat diseases. A correlation exists between the consumption of a diet high in saturated fats and the development of heart disease and hypertension. It is advisable to promote the consumption of healthy fats, such as olive oil, rice bran oil, and mustard oil, as an integral component of every meal, with a simultaneous avoidance of trans fats commonly present in fast food and fried foods.

"To optimize the efficacy of this dietary regimen, kindly take into consideration the ensuing recommendations:

A decrease in blood pressure can be achieved through a reduction in the consumption of alcoholic beverages.

Consequently, it is recommended to exercise moderation when consuming alcohol.

Aerobic exercise and adherence to the DASH diet contribute to a more rapid reduction in blood pressure.

Examine the nutritional information on food packaging to identify products with limited sodium content.

Despite maintaining a well-rounded dietary regimen, the presence of stress can lead to an increase in blood pressure. Engaging in practices such as meditation, yoga, and additional stress-alleviating activities can effectively contribute to the maintenance of optimal blood pressure.

Insomnia leads to an elevation in blood pressure. Consequently, maintaining a regular sleep duration of 7-8 hours per night can contribute to the regulation of your blood pressure.

Ceasing the habit of smoking will lead to a decrease in your blood pressure.

Please adhere to the recommended dosage instructions of your prescribed medication.

Please adhere to a maximum daily salt intake of one teaspoon.

Altering one's lifestyle necessitates effort. Attending to one's well-being necessitates a sustained dedication over an extended duration. Implementing gradual, incremental enhancements will result in more prompt and favorable outcomes compared to executing drastic, comprehensive alterations and potentially experiencing a decline in motivation.

It is highly advisable to seek guidance from a registered dietitian prior to commencing the DASH diet, in order to establish an individualized plan that caters to your specific dietary requirements.

Salad Composed Of Vegetables And Ham

Ingredients:

- ¼ cup onion, chopped
- ½ cup nonfat yogurt
- 1 tbsp sugar
- 1 tsp vinegar
- 1 cup ham, cooked
- 1 cup broccoli, chopped
- 1 carrot, peeled, diced
- 2 stalks celery, sliced thin

Directions:

1. Take chopped broccoli, diced carrots, celery, onion, and ham and mix in a large bowl.

2. In separate bowl, mix together yogurt with sugar and vinegar.
3. Combine the ingredients from each bowl and incorporate thoroughly. Enjoy.

Dietary Recommendations For Consumption And Avoidance Under The Dash Diet

Culinary discussions are widely revered among individuals. When food is mentioned, it often elicits a smile from most individuals, as it possesses an inherent charm that stimulates both the mind and the body, engendering a sense of exhilaration. Nutrition serves as an essential requirement for everyday existence, an indispensable element for sustenance that should ideally be consumed at a minimum frequency of three meals per day. There is a plethora of subjects to be addressed when considering food based on specific principles. Whether it is a matter of well-being, physical vitality, pleasantness, or adversity. This section will be dedicated to elucidating the guidelines and precautions pertaining to food consumption, including recommended dietary choices and those that should be avoided.

Dining Options" or "Culinary Choices

Lipids

These are high-calorie foods that should be carefully monitored to avoid excessive consumption. Excessive consumption of fats inevitably leads to the outcome of obesity. In addition, obesity carries substantial risks and poses a significant danger. It serves as a contributing factor to various illnesses.

Some exemplars of lipid-laden sustenance encompass:

Yogurt emulsion

Biscuits

Cakes

Deep-fried dishes

Butter and margarine in bread

It is generally recommended to consume fats in modest quantities in order to promote physical well-being.

Proteins

Proteins are an essential food group that holds significant importance within the body, as they fulfill a pivotal role in facilitating various internal functions such as overseeing the regulation of body and organ tissues. Proteins should constitute the predominant source of nutrition on the menu. They contribute to the growth and strengthening of the skeletal and muscular systems, which are indispensable for a multitude of everyday physical engagements. The majority of proteins are present in animal-derived food items.

There are four compelling rationales for incorporating protein into your dietary regimen:

a) They are engaged in the process of repairing bodily tissues.

b) They assist in combating diseases within the body through the actions of white blood cells.

c) They play a pivotal role in facilitating the majority of the body's transportation processes.

d) Adequate protein intake is crucial for optimal growth and development in infants, children, and pregnant women.

Some instances of protein-rich foods are as follows:

Canned baked legumes.

Chapatti

Meat

Fish
Eggs
Milk used in cereal
Legumes
Beef

Carbohydrates

These are foods abundant in molecules composed of three primary elements: carbon, hydrogen, and oxygen. On certain occasions, they are also denoted as starchy foods.

Some instances of carbohydrates include the following:

Bread
White and brown rice
Potatoes
Skinless chicken portions"

Fiber

In this category, the consumption of fiber-rich foods is of utmost significance and is often consumed in generous quantities. This food category is recommended by the physician to be consumed in substantial quantities. Based on contemporary research conducted across multiple scenarios, fiber has been found to offer numerous advantages. For example, it acts as a deterrent against the body becoming empty, thereby maintaining a higher level of fullness on a consistent basis. In addition, fiber is widely recognized for its capacity to mitigate the risk of diabetes and to decrease cholesterol levels within the body.

Below are instances of fiber:

Fruits

Vegetables

Nutritious morning meal with whole grain components

Nuts are a type of edible seeds or dry fruits that typically have a hard shell.

Whole grain brown rice

Dietary Restrictions for Weight Loss

Beverages high in sugar Sweetened beverages Drinks containing a significant amount of sugar Sugar-laden drinks

Confectionery bars.

Frozen dairy-based dessert.

Foods that have been subjected to deep-frying.

Adding cream to milk

Additional Types of Food to Avoid

Prepared meals for microwave consumption "Ready-to-heat food items

"Convenience foods designed for microwaving

The microwave is highly beneficial for a majority of individuals due to its ability to expedite cooking processes and significantly save time, particularly for individuals who prioritize the preparation of convenient meals. Well, that is good. It provides considerable assistance, nevertheless, the microwave is renowned for presenting significant concerns as well. For example, it can result in the development of diabetes or the observation that the food prepared lacks uniformity in its cooking.

Frankfurters

It is indeed accurate that they possess a high level of sweetness and palatability, making them a popular choice among individuals, particularly when engaging in sports or following physical exertion on the streets. Hot dogs can be classified as foods of minimal nutritional value that are high in fat content, potentially contributing to weight gain if appropriate measures are not implemented. The primary hazard associated with this is the inclusion of sodium, which serves no essential purpose within the human body.

Doughnuts

Doughnuts are an alternative confectionary that garners substantial admiration due to their delectable charm. Regrettably, it is a substantiated fact that these doughnuts are crafted utilizing genetically modified organisms (GMOs), which, when consumed excessively, have been linked to the development of cancer and even premature fatality due to arterial blockage.

Pizza

Pizza is at the top in the list of the world eaten junk food with the most deliveries in a day. Many individuals thoroughly enjoy ordering pizza when hosting gatherings at home, when entrusted with solitude by their parents, or when no other viable food options are readily available and hunger prevails. Pizza comprises various calorie-dense ingredients, making it advisable to cease consumption of this food as of today.

These are a few examples of the foods that you should exercise caution with and approach with a high level of seriousness. Should you choose to experiment with these methods, it is highly likely that you will experience an increase in body fat rather than achieve weight loss. Although these treats may appear innocuous due to their sweetness, they possess the ability to substantially contribute to caloric accumulation within the body. Rather than opting for those, you should choose alternatives that are less detrimental and have fewer or no calories. Consider integrating the following selection into your menu, and in the span of a month, you will witness a remarkable transformation in your physique.

Lean poultry, specifically chicken breast
Mashed potatoes.
Whole grain rice
The legumes with a green hue
Porcine Loin

The selection of meals is dictated by the time of day, categorized into three distinct periods: morning (breakfast), midday (lunch), and evening (supper).

Each specific time period has its own set of recommendations and, as advised by nutritionists, the ideal meal choice for lunch may not align with what is recommended for breakfast. Each time has its own appropriate dietary considerations. Some individuals may view consuming breakfast as discretionary, opting to forego the meal and instead indulge in a substantial lunch. Whilst there may not be inherent detriment in doing so, it remains true that all three categories of sustenance hold significant importance and should not be disregarded under any circumstances.

What would be suitable for consumption as a morning meal?

This particular meal has a historical association with improper consumption practices. Many individuals are not familiar with the correct dietary regimen for breakfast due to their lack of accustomed eating habits. Rest assured, I will provide assistance in that matter. Presented below are a selection of suitable options commonly recommended for consumption during breakfast time.

Based on extensive research findings, eggs have emerged as a highly favored breakfast choice and are recognized for their ability to effectively regulate blood sugar levels, particularly through the consumption of egg yolks.

Greek yogurt, renowned for its high protein content, serves as a potent energy source for the body. Yogurt is predominantly favored due to its ability to provide sustained satiety, ensuring a longer duration before experiencing hunger pangs once more.

Coffee - individuals who frequently or extensively engage in office work tend to favor coffee over tea, primarily due to its reputation for promoting alertness and fostering a cheerful disposition.

Nuts - not only do they possess a pleasant and palatable quality, but they also hold significant significance in the realm of regulating body weight, thereby mitigating the risk of developing obesity.

What would be an appropriate choice for today's midday meal?

There are those who posit that breakfast holds a greater significance compared to lunch, while others contend that the reverse is true. I believe it is important to not be deceived by others' opinions. Lunch holds significant importance within the overall meal structure, serving as a crucial sustenance to carry you through the afternoon with satiety. Lunch yields greater effectiveness, particularly when consumed appropriately and in appropriate portions.

Presented below are a selection of top choices to be deliberated for your midday repast.
Produce" or "horticultural edibles
Sandwich
Poultry-based salad
Chips
The legumes of the color black
Potatoes
The midday meal holds significance in multiple respects. As an illustration, the midday meal holds significance as it serves to elevate blood glucose levels throughout the day, thereby fostering

heightened focus and attentiveness throughout the remainder of the afternoon. It is imperative that individuals who approach lunchtime with a lackadaisical attitude understand the gravity of the situation, as neglecting this crucial meal can lead to significant repercussions, particularly if one is engaged in professional work or pursuing academics. This phenomenon arises due to the fact that skipping lunch increases the likelihood of being distracted and lacking focus during classes, ultimately resulting in subpar performance by the end of the day.

What shall we partake in for our evening meal?

Dinner constitutes one of the most demanding periods within the meal arrangement, posing significant challenges for many individuals, particularly unmarried individuals residing independently. These individuals constitute the group of individuals who depart for work in the morning and come back to their dwellings late at night, physically and mentally fatigued. At this juncture, the mind is predominantly fatigued and desires nothing more than for one to proceed to the shower, indulge in a rejuvenating warm bath, and retire until the following day. This is a common occurrence among a majority of workers, particularly those who earn low wages and bear the burden of long working hours. Listed below are several uncomplicated dishes that can be easily prepared for your evening meal, requiring minimal cooking time before being served.

Spaghetti

Casserole made from braised beef with vegetables in a rich broth.

Tuna combined with avocado

Chicken casserole

eggs prepared in a scrambled fashion

Broccoli

These are a selection of expeditious meal options to be prepared swiftly before retiring for the evening. Alternatively, if time permits, one may consider indulging in a dish comprised of brown rice, sautéed meat, or a choice of fish.

The subsequent suggestions may assist you in adapting to the DASH lifestyle:

- Prioritize the augmentation of vegetable consumption initially. Substitute starchy side dishes during the midday meal and include a portion of vegetables as an alternative. Ultimately, adhere to the same protocol during the evening meal.

- Ensure that fresh cut fruit is readily available as a substitute for sugary treats.

- Enhance your consumption of fat-free and low-fat dairy products to three servings per day.

- Exercise portion restraint when consuming protein. Constrain the consumption of meat, seafood, or poultry to three ounces per meal, equivalent to the approximate dimensions of a standard deck of cards.

- Please remove the salt dispenser from both the dining table and your food preparation area. Engage in trials with spice blends that are devoid of sodium as an alternative.

Modifications

Given that there are no "mandatory" food items specified in this plan, individuals who adhere to specific diets should be able to consume according to the DASH guidelines. As an illustration, individuals adhering to a gluten-free dietary regimen have the option to select grains that are considered safe, such as buckwheat or quinoa.

Individuals practicing veganism and vegetarianism can also adhere to the dietary principles outlined by DASH. In point of fact, the consumption of vegetarian meals is encouraged. Dairy consumption is not mandatory according to the implemented guidelines, and certain investigations9 have even posited that non-diary constituents of the dietary regimen (as opposed to milk products) are accountable for the associated health advantages.

In conclusion, for individuals who desire to increase their fat intake, there exists some evidence suggesting that following a higher fat variation of the DASH plan can potentially yield equivalent health advantages.

A study conducted in 2016 and published in the American Journal of Clinical Nutrition revealed that a higher fat variation of the DASH diet yielded comparable reductions in blood pressure when compared to the conventional DASH diet, while avoiding a significant increase in LDL cholesterol levels. In the study, individuals who adhered to the higher fat variant of the diet opted for full-fat dairy products instead of low-fat or nonfat dairy alternatives. They also decreased their sugar intake by limiting their consumption of fruit juice.

If you opt to adhere to the DASH diet for health-related purposes and wish to make alterations, it is advisable to consult your healthcare provider regarding the potential impact of your desired modifications on your health. At times, making modifications to one's dietary regimen can assist in adhering to the prescribed eating plan, however, it is advisable to seek the guidance of a healthcare professional to ensure the alignment of these adjustments with one's overarching health objectives.

The Advantages and Disadvantages of the DASH Diet
Pros

- Evidence-based health benefits

- Accessible

- Flexible

- Nutritional balance

- Developed with the purpose of promoting lifelong well-being

- Supported by prominent health organizations

Cons

- Hard to maintain

- No convenience foods

- No organized support

- Requires extensive food monitoring

- This product is not intended for the purpose of facilitating weight loss.

- May not be suitable for all individuals.

Pros

Evidence-Based Health Benefits

Extensive research has been conducted on the DASH diet. The original study that introduced the dietary regimen was published in 1997. It revealed that the implementation of this eating plan proved effective in reducing elevated blood pressure levels for individuals with normal blood pressure. Furthermore, it demonstrated even greater reduction in individuals diagnosed with hypertension.

After the introduction of the initial study, subsequent research has validated the aforementioned findings. According to a study conducted in 2016, it was determined that the DASH dietary approach may be the most effective means of reducing blood pressure in hypertensive and pre-hypertensive patients when considering high-quality evidence.

Furthermore, individuals adhering to the dietary regimen can anticipate additional health advantages. Additional studies have indicated that the DASH diet effectively decreases levels of LDL cholesterol and potentially enhances other factors contributing to cardiovascular risk. The DASH diet has demonstrated efficacy as a viable management approach for diabetes, and research findings have even indicated that adherence to the DASH diet may contribute to a reduction in the likelihood of developing gout among males.

In addition to supporting research on the DASH diet, numerous studies consistently indicate that decreasing sugar consumption, eliminating highly processed foods with high sodium content, and increasing fruit and vegetable intake contribute to a diverse array of health advantages.

Accessible

The food advocated by the DASH diet is readily available in nearly any supermarket. No rare ingredients, essential foods, supplements, or subscriptions are necessary to adhere to the program.

Furthermore, in contrast to commercially available diet plans, all the necessary information for this program can be accessed online at no cost. The National Institutes of Health offers a diverse array of resources, which encompass a comprehensive manual on suggested servings, meal plans, recommendations for sodium intake, guides on caloric intake, informational pamphlets, and culinary recipes.

There are also countless cookbooks, websites, and smartphone apps dedicated to this eating style. Furthermore, due to extensive research and widespread endorsement within the medical community, it is highly probable that your healthcare provider will be acquainted with this particular diet. Therefore, if you have any inquiries regarding whether or not to adhere to the proposed strategy, they are likely skilled in providing guidance.

Flexible

Dietary plans following the Dietary Approaches to Stop Hypertension (DASH) guidelines are accessible in diverse caloric options in order to cater to individuals of varying gender and physical exertion levels.1 Determining the appropriate energy consumption can be easily accomplished by referring to the online charts provided by the National Institutes of Health (NIH).

Moreover, individuals adhering to specific dietary restrictions can adopt the Dietary Approaches to Stop Hypertension (DASH) eating plan. Individuals adhering to a vegetarian or vegan lifestyle will discover that this plan aligns seamlessly with their dietary preferences, as the consumption of grains, fruits, and vegetables is highly emphasized. Those individuals who adhere to a gluten-free diet can sustain their dietary regimen by opting for permissible grains such as buckwheat and quinoa. Individuals adhering to a kosher or Halal diet can select food options that comply with the respective dietary requirements and continue to adhere to the prescribed plan.

Nutritional Balance

While many diets necessitate consumers to make drastic adjustments to their macronutrient intake, such as low-carb or low-fat diets, or severely restrict calories, the DASH diet adheres to the nutritional guidelines set forth by the USDA.

As an illustration, if you were to follow the DASH diet, approximately 55% of your daily calorie intake would consist of carbohydrates. The United States Department of Agriculture (USDA) advises a range of 45% to 65% of your total caloric intake to be derived from carbohydrates.

As per the guidelines provided by the United States Department of Agriculture (USDA), it is recommended that 20% to 35% of your caloric intake should be derived from fats, with less than 10% of those calories coming from saturated fats. Similarly, on the DASH diet, it is advised that no more than 27% of your caloric intake should come from fats, and a maximum of 6% of those calories should be sourced from saturated fats.

By adhering to the program, you should also be capable of achieving your recommended consumption of other crucial nutrients, including protein, fiber, and calcium.8

Lifelong Wellness

The DASH diet is considered a long-term, sustainable approach rather than a temporary program. The dietary regimen is structured to be a lifelong commitment.

Guidelines are offered to assist individuals adhering to a conventional American diet in gradually transitioning towards reduced consumption of red meat, processed foods, while increasing their intake of fruits and vegetables. Modifications are implemented in a gradual manner to foster adherence.

As an illustration, the experts in the field of DASH recommend a reduction in sodium intake to 2,300 milligrams per day before endeavoring to further decrease it to 1,500 milligrams—an extent that could potentially procure enhanced health advantages for certain individuals. Furthermore, there is no arduous initial phase where the intake of calories or daily carbohydrates is drastically reduced.

Supported by Prominent Health Associations" or "Endorsed by Leading Healthcare Institutions

The DASH diet has received endorsement from several reputable institutions such as the National Institutes of Health, National Heart, Lung, and Blood Institute, the American Heart Association, the American Diabetes Association, the USDA, as well as esteemed medical institutions including the Mayo Clinic and the Cleveland Clinic. Furthermore, it has been ranked as the second best overall diet according to U.S. News and World Report.

Cons

Hard to Maintain

Individuals who adhere to a conventional American dietary pattern might encounter difficulties when attempting to adapt to the DASH regimen. The program advises a reduction in your salt consumption to 2,300 milligrams of sodium per day and possibly down to as low as 1,500 milligrams per day.

As per the statistics provided by the Centers for Disease Control, the typical sodium intake of the average American amounts to 3,400 milligrams per day. A significant proportion of the sodium we consume is derived from extensively processed food products, which are limited within the restrictions imposed by the DASH dietary regimen.

Even if one refrains from consuming processed food, relinquishing the habitual use of the salt shaker proves to be challenging for numerous individuals.

Due to this rationale, as well as various other factors, adhering to the DASH diet can prove to be demanding. A research endeavor exploring adherence to the DASH diet revealed challenges in maintaining compliance among individuals, thus indicating a requirement for additional interventions beyond counseling to foster long-term adherence.

Furthermore, scholars have conducted examinations on the consumption of dietary fat within the Dietary Approaches to Stop Hypertension (DASH) regimen, postulating that incorporating higher levels of fat into the diet could potentially enhance adherence to the program.

In a certain study, individuals adhered to a diet that had higher fat content and opted for full-fat dairy products rather than low-fat or nonfat options. Additionally, they reduced their sugar intake by limiting their consumption of fruit juice. The study revealed that the elevated fat variant of the DASH diet effectively decreased blood pressure to a similar degree as the conventional DASH diet without significantly elevating LDL cholesterol levels.

Exquisite Handcrafted Greek-Inspired Yogurt

Ingredients:

½ cup of live yogurt culture (or regular plain yogurt)

Thermometer

Cheesecloth for straining

Small blanket

1 cup of powdered milk (this is optional but does make the yogurt thicker)

1/2 gallon

2 percent milk

Directions:

Commence the process of adding milk into the slow cooker and proceed to incorporate powdered milk while stirring. Subject the substance to elevated temperatures until it attains a measure of 180 degrees Fahrenheit, which will typically require approximately one to two hours. Subsequently, proceed to disengage the slow cooker and proceed with the process of cooling the milk to a temperature of 110 degrees Fahrenheit. Subsequently, it is advised to incorporate the live yogurt culture and thoroughly blend all ingredients until they are fully combined. Disable the slow cooker and envelop it with a blanket to preserve the heat. Allow to rest undisturbed for a duration of 8 hours. At this juncture, kindly remove the cover of the slow cooker and add a generous amount of Greek-style yogurt to the mixture. To separate the whey, or the liquid component of the yogurt, it is advisable to utilize a colander lined with multiple layers of cheesecloth, positioning it atop a substantial bowl. Blend the yogurt with the colander and allow it to undergo the process of drainage in the refrigerator for a duration of a few hours. It is advised to extract it exclusively upon achieving the desired consistency. Your delectable Hellenic yogurt is now prepared. Please proceed with transferring the yogurt into mason jars (or alternative containers) and proceed to store it in the refrigerator for a duration of 8 days.

There exist numerous factors that could contribute to individuals' inclination to experiment with the DASH Diet. An individual may aspire to shed weight, adopt a more nutritious dietary regimen, reduce their blood pressure, or decrease their cholesterol levels. Moreover, a subset of individuals perceive heightened levels of energy as a consequence of adhering to the DASH Diet, owing to its comparatively lower sugar content in comparison to alternative dietary regimens. Regardless of the underlying motivation for desiring to adopt the DASH Diet, it is important to acknowledge that certain difficulties may arise when embarking upon such a regimen.

An obstacle that arises when attempting to implement this plan is acquiring knowledge about the selection and timing of meals throughout the day. The DASH Diet is structured around the consumption of protein-rich foods while restricting the intake of sugars. These particular food options are generally recommended for the majority of individuals. However, adherents of the DASH Diet are required to devise alternative methods of incorporating these foods into their meals, as the diet restricts the consumption of certain items throughout the entire day.

While the DASH Diet does offer some leeway in determining which days one can consume specific types of foods, adhering to this regimen on a daily basis remains quite challenging. To determine appropriate timing and portion sizes of meals throughout the day, familiarizing oneself with fundamental principles will assist in adhering to a suitable caloric intake.

To commence with, the DASH Diet is characterized by its considerable protein content. In order to adhere to your daily caloric intake, it will be necessary for you to consume a substantial amount of protein. This may be difficult because not everyone likes to eat certain kinds of foods; however, there are some different ways that you can convert foods into proteins for the DASH Diet.

What are the primary objectives that they will seek to achieve through this dietary regimen?

A primary objective of this dietary plan is to facilitate the achievement and sustenance of an optimal body weight, as engaging in prolonged periods of very-low-calorie regimens, wherein individuals consume between 1,600–2,400 calories daily, can lead to numerous adverse health ramifications. This can result in malnutrition, as well as a significant deficiency in vital nutrients like dietary fiber, folate, zinc, and vitamin D.

There is considerable ongoing discourse pertaining to the optimal dietary regimen for weight loss, as certain individuals advocate for carbohydrate consumption while others emphasize the significance of fat intake. The primary objective of this diet regimen is to facilitate weight reduction while ensuring sustenance, thereby enabling a lasting, non-depriving approach to weight management. Extensive research spanning a decade has been conducted by scientists, yielding profound insights that strongly suggest the effectiveness of this dietary regimen for individuals seeking weight loss.

As an illustration, it is worth noting that a comprehensively conducted scientific review meticulously analyzed 15 distinct research studies on the DASH Diet over a span of 6 years. It was determined that the utilization of the DASH Diet yielded positive results in aiding weight reduction, while simultaneously facilitating the management of individuals' blood pressure and blood cholesterol levels. In particular, the researchers discovered that the DASH Diet yielded positive outcomes with regard to enhancing lipid profile, reducing blood pressure, and facilitating weight reduction. Additionally, they discovered that implementing this dietary regimen proved to be a financially viable approach in facilitating individuals' overall well-being. The safety and effectiveness of the DASH Diet have been substantiated over an extended duration, an attribute that is notably uncommon among diets of comparable popularity.

An additional research study demonstrated that implementation of the DASH Diet resulted in notable reduction in body weight among individuals categorized as obese, without any reported incidences of adverse effects or negative responses. The aforementioned research was disseminated in 2006 within the pages of the Journal of the American Medical Association (JAMA).

Advantages of the DASH Diet

In contemporary times, a multitude of diets favoring diverse food categories have gained popularity, yet a significant portion of individuals encounter challenges in adhering to these diets within their daily routines. Obtaining proper nourishment and weight management can pose challenges in the absence of professional dietary guidance, as it necessitates consumption of a diverse range of nutritious foods. This explains the recent surge in popularity of the DASH Diet.

DASH represents the abbreviation for "Diabetes, Atherosclerosis, Hypertension, and Heart Attack Prevention," although its advantages surpass the scope of solely addressing these medical conditions. It aids individuals in mitigating health conditions such as cancer, obesity, anemia, and osteoporosis. The DASH Diet comprises an assortment of fruits, vegetables, whole grains, lean meats, low-fat dairy products, and healthy fats.

An Examination of the Advantages of the DASH Diet

The primary advantage of this dietary regimen, as its nomenclature suggests, lies in its capacity to enhance personal well-being and safeguard against the onset of chronic conditions such as diabetes, atherosclerosis, and hypertension. This dietary plan has been specifically devised to cater to individuals with these conditions, however, it is applicable to anyone seeking to enhance their overall well-being.

The second advantage lies in the renowned DASH Diet weight loss regimen, which facilitates speedy and effective weight reduction, surpassing the efficacy of alternative diets available in the market. The crux lies in its emphasis on holistic nutrition as opposed to mere weight loss. If you adhere to this program for a duration of 12 consecutive weeks, notable improvements in both your physical appearance and overall well-being will be evident.

The third advantage of adhering to this dietary plan is its potential to decrease the likelihood of developing blood clots and cardiovascular ailments. Adopting a nutritious diet and engaging in consistent physical activity contribute to the prevention of ailments like hypertension, myocardial infarction, and cerebrovascular accident.

The fourth advantage entails the capacity to avert the occurrences of cancer, obesity, anemia, and osteoporosis. These conditions are associated with elevated cholesterol levels, which also serve as a contributing factor for various health complications. Foods such as fish, poultry, nuts, and legumes exhibit efficacy in mitigating cholesterol levels. By integrating these diverse food groups into your daily dietary regimen, you will markedly enhance your overall well-being, often without conscious awareness.

The fifth advantage lies in its sustainable approach, which actively encourages the cultivation of healthy dietary practices. It aids in acquiring the ability to consume food in a manner that enhances one's emotional well-being, cognitive abilities, and drive. The essential nutrients can be found in the diet choices you make. Not only is it cost-effective, but it also offers practicality due to its user-friendly nature that allows for convenient usage both in domestic settings and while on the go.

The Food Program

The DASH Nutritional Protocol

The DASH diet does not solely concentrate on sodium; it also restricts various forms and types of food. It additionally places significant importance on the specified quantity of food per portion. It establishes a designated space or container for sustenance throughout the day, wherein your daily consumption is restricted to a level that promotes dietary equilibrium. Achieving such control becomes challenging in the absence of adherence to the DASH diet, as this dietary regimen provides a comprehensive guide to optimal nutritional strategies. It has been constructed with the intention of altering our perspectives on food and transforming our consumption habits. It primarily operates utilizing two distinct mechanisms. Initially, it governs the calibre of the repast, and furthermore, it dictates the magnitude of the repast. Through the implementation of these practices, one can attain heightened health advantages that surpass the guarantees of any other dietary regimen. The food is initially sorted into distinct classifications, such as fruits, vegetables, whole grains, legumes, nuts, meat, or dairy. Subsequently, one must analyze the health ramifications inherent to each category, and it is advised to take into account their proportion in a solitary meal or serving.

Scientifically Proven Advantages of the DASH Diet

Early research on the significance of the DASH Diet was conducted by the National Institute of Health in the United States. Scientists were cognizant of the consequences of such a dietary regime, yet they required empirical evidence to bolster their assertion. Therefore, three distinct dietary regimens were formulated to assess the effects. The strategy that demonstrated the highest quantity of fruits, vegetables, beans, and non-fat dairy products proved to be the most efficacious in reducing diastolic and systolic blood pressures by 3 mmHg and 6 mmHg, correspondingly. While the DASH diet imposes restrictions on specific food items, it also emphasizes the importance of moderating calorie intake. It maintains a daily caloric consumption ranging from 1600 to 3100. This datum assumes greater significance when confronted with the issue of obesity. The DASH diet, through its adherence to the Optimal Macronutrient Intake Trial for heart health, achieved commendable results in decreasing regular fat consumption and effectively mitigating a variety of cardiovascular ailments.

It represents a sustainable and enduring solution.

Individuals with hypertension may not always rely on medications as a sustainable approach for maintaining long-term health stability. Regardless of the efficacy of the medications, they are not devoid of adverse effects. The adoption of dietary and lifestyle modifications can offer a sustained therapeutic solution coupled with proactive preventive measures. Hypertension is a chronic condition, with long-term implications, that remains persistent once it has been diagnosed, causing individuals to be indefinitely affected by this health issue. It is not a question of mere days; rather, it pertains to the entirety of their lifespan. Hence, solely adopting a dietary regimen is the key to mitigating high blood pressure and its corresponding complications.

Aids in the Management of Type 2 Diabetes

In order to comprehend the correlation between the DASH diet and diabetes, it is imperative to delve into the underlying factors contributing to Type 2 Diabetes. Consuming food with a high caloric content or experiencing weight gain are both factors that contribute to the body developing resistance to insulin. When you cross off both those factors, it becomes easier to control Types 2 Diabetes. The DASH diet effectively addresses and regulates both of these factors. To begin with, by means of its regulated serving methodology, and furthermore, by promoting the reduction of obesity. It enhances the body's insulin sensitivity, thereby mitigating the potential hazards associated with elevated blood glucose levels. Furthermore, by establishing a balanced dietary composition, the DASH diet establishes parameters for the consumption of carbohydrates, enabling the body to effectively control insulin secretion and perform its physiological processes in the absence of excessive carbohydrate intake.

Ten Compelling Factors Supporting the Efficacy of the DASH Diet

When discussing the DASH diet from a practical standpoint, one can observe its efficacy as a dietary approach. In addition to an abundance of research and experimentation, the primary motivations behind individuals' exploration of this dietary regimen lie in its distinctive attributes. It induces a sense of comfort and convenience, thereby fostering user acceptance of its established protocols and guidelines. Below are several justifications as to why the DASH Diet effectively yields exceptional outcomes:

1. Simple to Implement

The extensive array of choices encompassed by the DASH diet distinguishes it as a highly adaptable dietary approach applicable to all individuals. This is the underlying cause behind individuals' inclination to transition to it and effectively utilize its genuine health advantages. It facilitates enhanced adaptability for its users.

2. Promotes Exercise

It surpasses all other factors in effectiveness due to its comprehensive approach, which places equal emphasis on dietary intake, daily exercise, and routine physical activities. This is the underlying factor behind its ability to yield immediate, observable outcomes.

3. All Inclusive

With some restrictions in place, this Diet has incorporated each food item into its repertoire with certain adjustments. It aptly provides concise directions regarding the recommended practices and prohibitions for all constituents, safeguarding us from the consumption of detrimental substances detrimental to bodily well-being.

4. A method of achieving a state of equilibrium

One of the primary benefits it offers is its ability to uphold equilibrium in our dietary habits, daily regimen, caloric consumption, and nutritional nourishment.

5. Satisfactory Assessment of Energy Intake

Each meal that we intend to have following the DASH diet has been pre-determined and adjusted in accordance with calorie counts. We can conveniently monitor the daily caloric consumption and subsequently impose restrictions by eliminating specific food items.

6. Enforces Restriction on Unhealthy Food

The DASH diet recommends incorporating a greater quantity of organic and fresh produce while discouraging the consumption of processed food and unhealthy items found in stores. Thus, it fosters improved dietary practices among the users.

7. Dedicated to Proactive Measures

While the efficacy of this remedy has been validated for numerous ailments, it is commonly referred to as a proactive measure.

8. Gradual but Steady Transformations

The dietary plan is characterized by a moderate level of restriction and supports a gradual progression towards attaining optimal health. You have the flexibility to establish your desired targets on a daily, weekly, or monthly basis according to your convenience.

9. Effects over the long term.

The outcomes of the DASH diet are not only remarkable, but they also exhibit prolonged efficacy. The rate of progress is deemed to be sluggish, yet the impact is enduring.

10. Accelerates Metabolism

The DASH diet, known for its emphasis on overall wellness, possesses the capacity to stimulate and enhance our metabolic activity, thereby facilitating optimal bodily functioning.

Cranberry Orange Ground Sausage Discs

Ingredients:

- 2 tbsp minced, dried cranberries
- Zest of 1 orange
- ½ tsp red pepper flakes

- ¼ tsp black pepper
- 1 tsp fennel seeds
- a pinch of kosher salt
- ½ tsp thyme
- ⅓ cup no-added-sugar orange juice
- ½ tbsp brown sugar or honey
- 1 lb ground turkey

Directions:

Pulverize the fennel seeds and salt using a mortar and pestle. Incorporate the powdered spices along with thyme, black pepper, and red pepper flakes.

Incorporate the turkey, brown sugar, cranberries, minced garlic, orange zest, and freshly squeezed orange juice in a sizable mixing bowl. Incorporate the spices into the mixture, followed by shaping it into patties measuring ¼ cup each.

Allow the patties to rest in the refrigerator for a duration of 1 hour, in order to achieve a firmer consistency. Prepare the patties by cooking them on a stovetop pan or griddle set to medium heat, allowing each side to achieve a lightly golden brown appearance. Serve promptly without delay. In the event of preparation in advance, it is advised to freeze the patties by individually placing them on sheets of waxed paper until they are completely solidified. Next, proceed to carefully transfer the frozen patties into a hermetically sealed receptacle within the freezing compartment.

To present, arrange the sausage patties delicately on a split, wholesome whole wheat English muffin or alternatively, a tortilla with reduced sodium content.

Grapefruit Avocado Salad

Ingredients:

- 1 tablespoon honey
- Coriander leaves
- 1 tbsp peeled pumpkin seeds
- Salt pepper
- 2 grapefruits
- 1 ripe avocado
- 100g lamb's lettuce
- 1 spring onion
- ¼ LEMON
- 1 - 2 tablespoons of olive oil

Preparation:

Remove the peel of the grapefruits, including the pith, and proceed to divide them into smaller sections. Please ensure that the juice from the grapefruit is gathered in a receptacle. Proceed to meticulously peel and finely slice the avocado. Proceed to drizzle a portion of the grapefruit juice onto the slices of avocado. Dice the spring onions and transfer them into a bowl along with the lamb's lettuce, grapefruits, and avocado. Incorporate the olive oil, honey, and a quantity equivalent to 2 teaspoons of the lemon juice to create a dressing. Accurately season with salt and pepper and subsequently incorporate the crushed pumpkin seeds. Combine the dressing with the salad and garnish using the coriander leaves.

Peach Cobbler

Ingredients

- 1 1/2 cups of brown sugar
- 2 large peeled peaches, sliced
- 1 cup of all-purpose flour
- 1 pinch of ground nutmeg
- 1/4 tsp of salt
- 3/4 cups of milk
- 2 cups of baking powder
- 1/2 cup of butter, melted

Instructions

Set the oven temperature to 375 degrees Fahrenheit prior to use.

Allow the butter to liquify in a container. Obtain an additional bowl and combine sugar and peaches within. Combine salt, sugar, nutmeg, flour, milk, and baking powder in separate containers. Blend the ingredients until a cohesive and seamless batter is achieved.

Place the batter into the dish where the butter was previously melted. Top with sugared peaches. Bake in the oven for approximately 50 minutes until golden.

Serve and enjoy.

www.ingramcontent.com/pod-product-compliance
Lightning Source LLC
Chambersburg PA
CBHW070030040426
42333CB00040B/1415